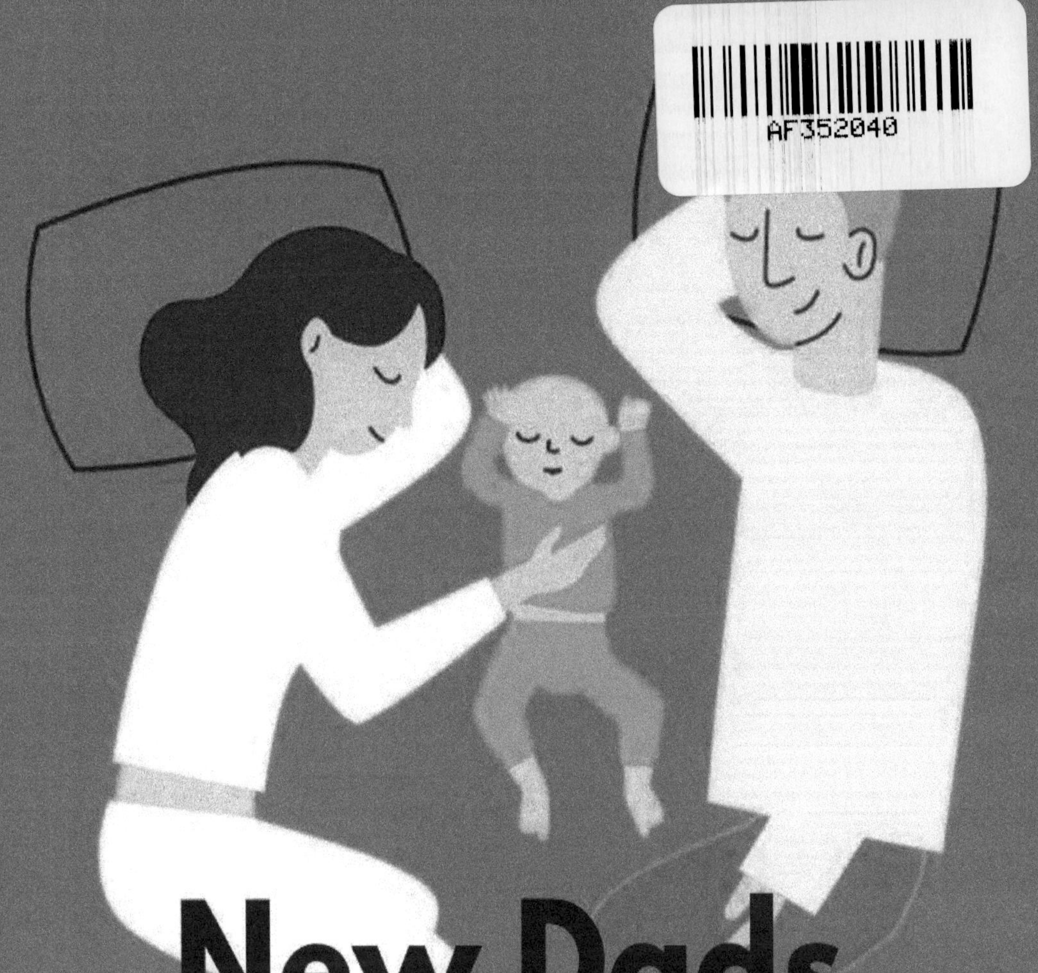

New Dads

A Basic Guide to Supporting the Breastfeeding Mother

Essential Knowledge for New Fathers, Mothers, Parents & Support People

Bed-sharing is a controversial topic. You must check with your pediatrician. La Leche league International has released, "Safe Sleep 7." This is a guide to safer bed-sharing.

H. Mae Scott IBCLC, IAIM, BA

Table of Contents

Dedication

This book is dedicated to my children, Lauren, Gary Jr, and Sam without whom I would not know the depth of a mothers love. To my grandchildren James, Chloe, and Benjamin, for bringing love and joy into my life. To my husband, Gary Sr. for his support. To my parents, Charlotte and Alan, and grandparents who treasured their children and guided me to be the parent I aspire to be. I would also like to thank my friends and family who have been so supportive during this process, Katherine, Brittany, Sandra, Gillian, Dominie, and Barbara.

One of the joys in life is having a wonderful partner, husband, or friend that you can count on during challenging times and then seeing the partnership or friendship grow. "This involves showing love, respect and active communication. It also means being supportive, trustworthy, and a caring partner. Prioritizing your relationship and personal growth are key elements."

-marriage.com

Forward

Breastfeeding isn't solely a mother's endeavor: It's a journey that requires steadfast support from partners, particularly new dads. "New Dads: A Basic Guide to Supporting the Breastfeeding Mother and Baby" recognized this essential role and offers a basic blueprint for dads to become proactive allies in the breastfeeding process.

This guide opens with a poignant acknowledgement of the pivotal role fathers play in facilitating successful breastfeeding. Backed by research from the National Institutes of Health, It emphasizes how a father's or partner's knowledge, attitude and involvement significantly impact the initiation and maintenance of breastfeeding. This sets the stage for an exploration of why dads' engagement is vital for both the mother's and the newborn's well-being.

What makes this guide invaluable is its holistic approach. It doesn't merely underscore the benefits of breastfeeding; it delves into the essential details, from the unique nutritional needs of breastfeeding mothers to the importance of advocating for their rights in various settings. It adeptly navigates through dietary considerations, highlighting the significance of a balanced diet while debunking myths surrounding certain food restrictions.

In essence, "New Dads: A Basic Guide to Supporting the Breastfeeding Mother and Baby" transcends the traditional confines of parenting literature. It's not just a guide: it's a manifesto for empowered fatherhood-a testament to the transformative impact dads can have in nurturing and sustaining breastfeeding journeys. With its blend of empathy, expertise and practicality, this guide is a must-read for every new dad embarking on the beautiful journey of parenthood.

Nicholas Neumann, Amazon Publishing Plus

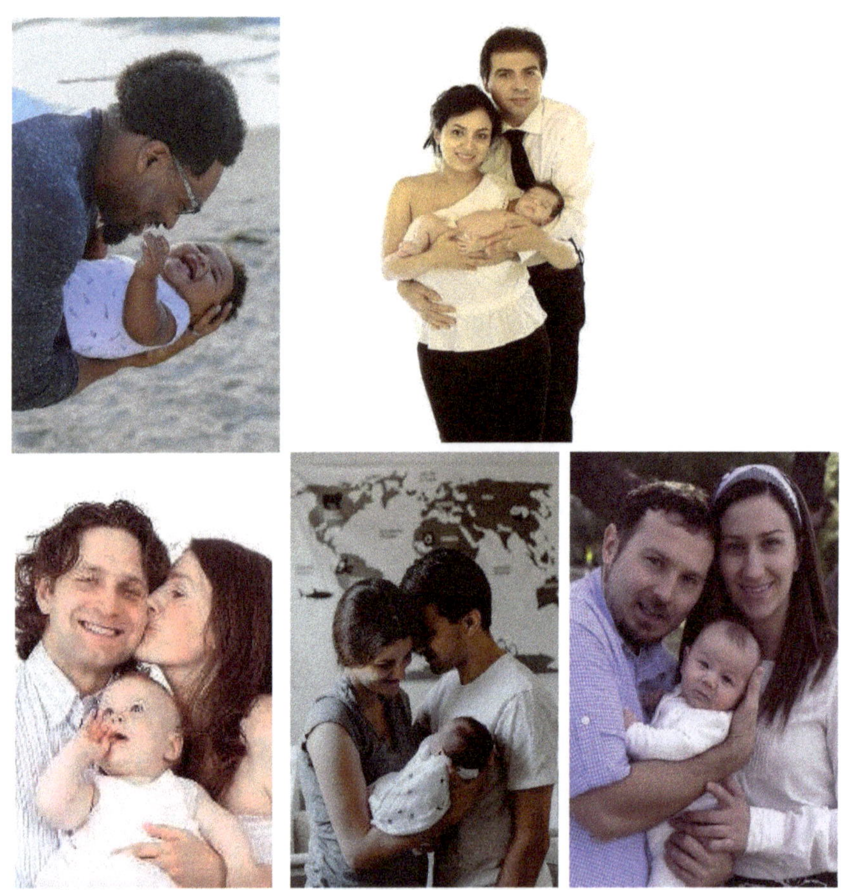

"The father of the baby is one of the most influential persons to the mother, and they can act as either key supporters or deterrents to breastfeeding."

https://Internationalbreastfeedingjournal,November 29, 2009

Introduction
Why Dads/Partners are Important to Successful Breastfeeding

Studies do show that Men and Partners are instrumental in working with moms to ensure the best possible outcome with breastfeeding. Many now want to have the knowledge they need to support their partner and baby in learning this important process. The National Institutes of Health says, "A father's knowledge and attitude are fundamental to beginning and maintaining breastfeeding. He has the most critical role in helping women with parenting and feeding their babies."

At this time, many new fathers are not taught how to support the baby's mother with the breastfeeding practice. This book is a basic introduction to what new fathers/dads/partners can do to be encouraging, knowledgeable and helpful. Couples can work together as a team to prepare for the best possible delivery, nutrition, caring and parenting for their children. If your decision is to breastfeed or try to breastfeed, encouragement and support from the partner can be critical in achieving success.

"Imagine that the world had created a new 'dream product' to feed and immunize everyone born on earth. Imagine also that it was available everywhere, required no storage or delivery, and helped (parents) and mothers plan their families and reduce the risk of cancer. Then imagine that the world refused to use it."

-Frank A. Oski

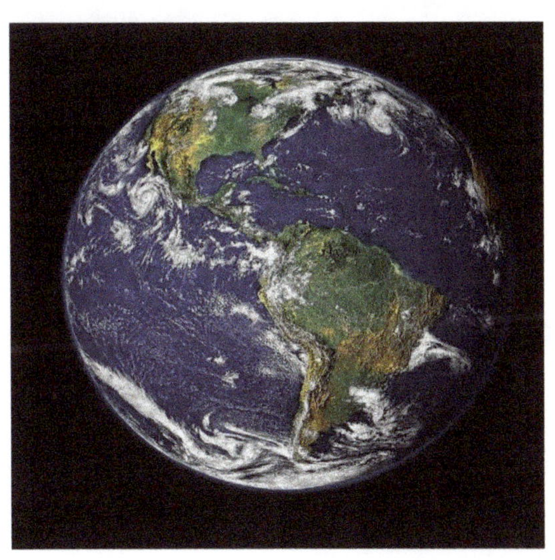

Chapter 1
The Benefits of Breastfeeding

Breastfeeding is a beautiful and natural process that not only provides essential nutrients and antibodies for your baby but offers numerous benefits for the mother as well. This process may be natural, but not always easy at first. Being an encouraging partner can be very beneficial to the mother learning to breastfeed. Understanding the benefits of breastfeeding for both mother and baby is crucial for new parents to fully appreciate the importance of this experience.

For the baby, breastfeeding is a vital source of nutrition that helps boost their immune system and protect them from illnesses. Breast milk is easily digested and contains the perfect balance of nutrients, ensuring optimal growth and development. Additionally, the act of breastfeeding promotes a strong bond between mother and baby, creating a sense of security and comfort for the infant.

Breastfeeding also provides numerous benefits for the mother. It helps reduce the possibility of certain cancers and stimulates the release of oxytocin, a hormone that promotes bonding and reduces stress. Breastfeeding can also aid in postpartum weight loss, as it burns extra calories and helps the uterus contract back to its pre-pregnancy size.

Human Breastmilk is a natural food made especially for a mother's child. It is specifically made for the mother's birth infant, for their age, gender and health status. It has the ability to continually change content for what the baby needs at that time and as they grow. For example, if a mother gets a cold, the baby will get the antibodies to help fight that cold.

The following pages will describe more of the benefits of breastfeeding for the mother and baby.

Breastmilk has MORE of the Good Things Babies Need
See for Yourself!

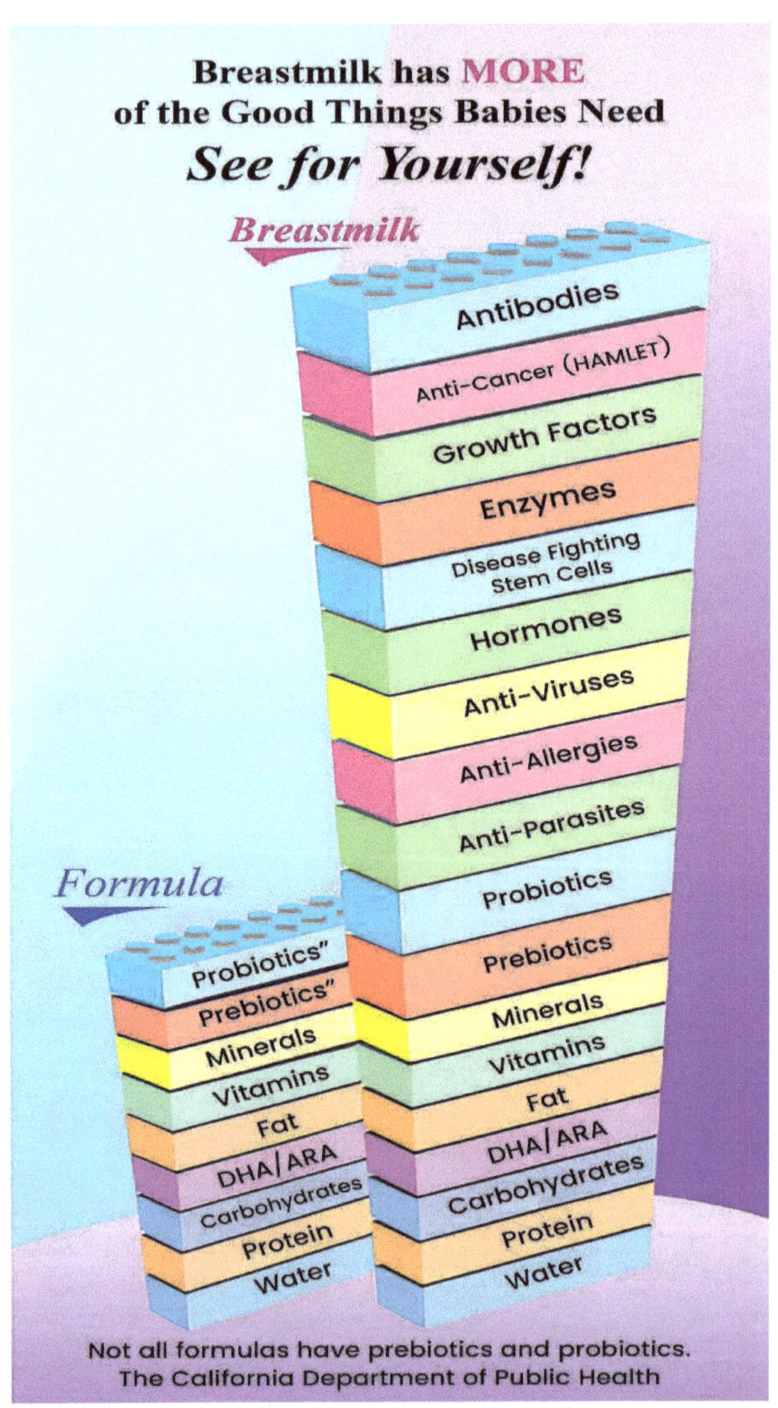

Benefits of Breastmilk for your baby

- Prevents Infections
- Less Illnesses
- Less trips to the pediatrician
- Lower risk for SIDS (Sudden Infant Death Syndrome)
- Less Diarrhea
- Less Digestive Conditions
- Lower Risk of Asthma
- Lower Risk of Obesity
- Lower Risk of Type 1 Diabetes
- Less Ear Infections
- Compared with formula, nutrients are better absorbed and used
- Best for brain growth and nervous system
- Eyes work better
- Helps build a Strong Immune System, and more......

cdc.gov.johnshopkinsmedicine.org, www.nichd.nih.gov

Breastfeeding and Jaw Development

"Breastfeeding is important to proper jaw development because it places beneficial orthopedic forces on the jaws during a rapid period of infant jaw growth. Breast suckling aids the proper development of the jaws, which form the gateway to the human airway. Bottle, pacifier and digit sucking deform jaws and airways."

https://pubmed.ncbi.nlm.nig.gov/11799699/

"Extensive research in the literature demonstrated that prolonged breastfeeding plays a crucial role in preventing the development of malocclusion (improper bite), enhancing the sagittal (vertical plane) growth of the mandible (lower jaw) and establishing proper occlusal (how upper and lower teeth come together) relationships by stimulating the facial muscles during lactation."

https://www.ncbi.nlm.nih.gov>pmc

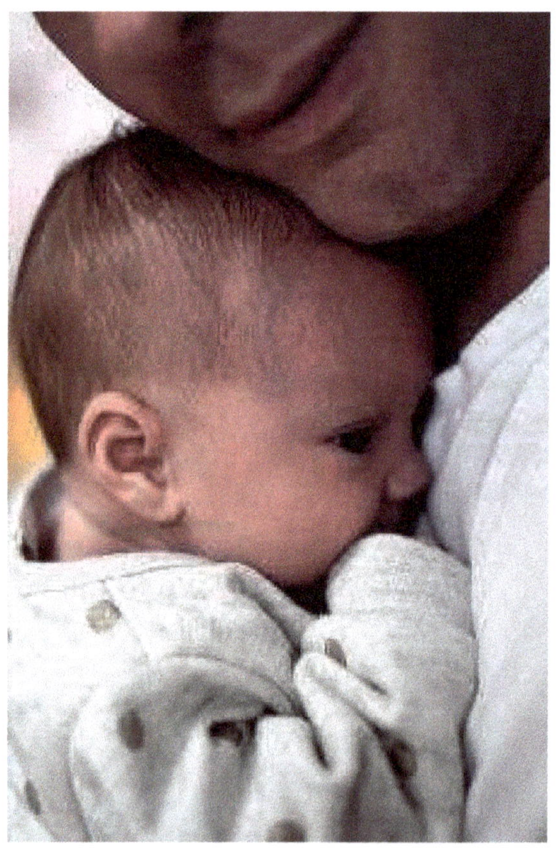

Benefits of Breastfeeding for the Mother

- Lose baby weight quicker
- Lower risk of developing breast and ovarian cancer, heart disease and osteoporosis
- Produces Oxytocin, the "feel good" hormone
- Oxytocin promotes healing, reduces stress, and helps uterus contract.
- May protect against postnatal depression
- Enhances bonding with baby
- Once established, is time saving
- Less sick days from work
- Milk is always the right temperature no or less bottle sterilizing

  cdc.gov,johnshopkinsmedicine.org,www.nichd.nih.gov

Many studies do show that breastmilk is the superior infant food choice, and is highly recommended. If Breastfeeding is not possible or adequate, Formula is an alternative substitute that intends to copy breastmilk as closely as possible.

Contraindications to Breastfeeding

There are rare times when breastfeeding is not recommended. Always check with your doctors and healthcare professionals for the most updated recommendations. As of February 6, 2024, the CDC recommends the following;

Infant Contraindications to Breastfeeding

- If the infant has classic galactosemia, a rare genetic metabolic disorder

Mother Contraindications to Breastfeeding

-If the mother has HIV and

a) are not on HIV treatment

b) are treated but not sustained viral suppression during pregnancy and after birth. Must check with your Doctors.

- T-cell lymphotropic virus types I and II
- If they are using illicit drugs, such as opioids or cocaine. If they discontinue and are on stable methadone or buprenorphine maintenance therapy, breastfeeding can resume with the Doctor's permission.
- If they have confirmed or suspected Ebola virus disease.

Mother needs to temporarily stop breastfeeding when

- They are infected with untreated brucellosis
- They are taking certain medications. Check with your doctors
- They are undergoing imaging with radiopharmaceuticals

- They have active herpes simplex virus with lesions on the breast. Can breastfeed on the unaffected breast if lesions on the affected side are covered completely
- They have mpox virus infection

Mothers should temporarily stop but can resume expressed breastmilk if;

- They have untreated, active TB. May resume after 2 weeks treated and the doctor confirms she is no longer contagious and says it is safe to breastfeed
- They have active chickenpox that developed between 5 days before birth and 2 days following delivery.

www.cdc.gov (http://www.cdc.gov)

"Mothers and babies form an inseparable biological and social unit; the health and nutrition of one group cannot be divorced from the health and nutrition of the other."

-World Health Organization

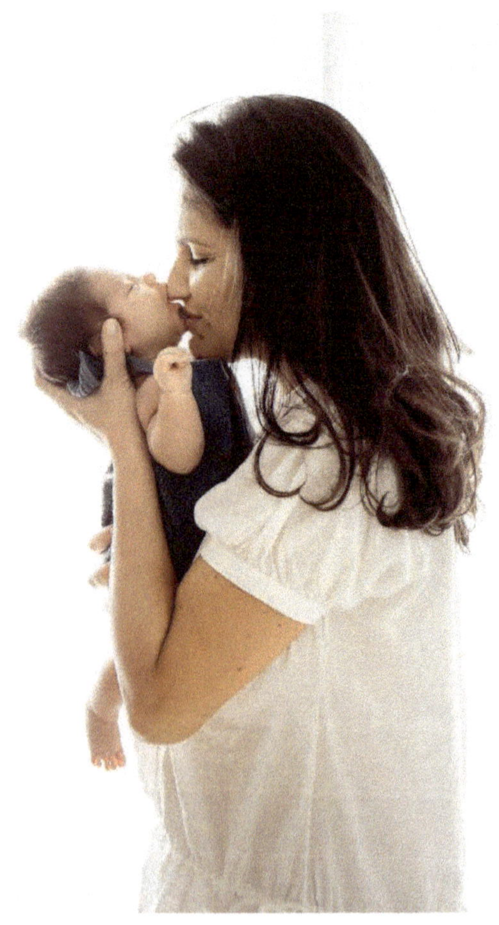

Chapter 2
Exploring the Nutritional Needs of a Breastfeeding Mother

A breastfeeding mother's nutritional needs are unique, as she requires additional calories and nutrients to support lactation. The Mayo Clinic suggests an additional 330 - 400 kcal per day for the lactating mother. It is important to encourage her to eat a balanced diet rich in fruits, vegetables, whole grains, lean proteins and healthy fats. Because of differing diets, your healthcare provider can advise you as to whether she needs to take any vitamins or supplements. Certain types of seafood should be limited or not eaten if there are high levels of Mercury in them. Swordfish, tuna, shark, king mackerel and tilefish have the highest levels of mercury. Caffeine can possibly affect the infant and should be limited. Not drinking alcohol is the safest option for lactating mothers. Drinking alcohol can decrease the infant's milk intake and can cause other issues. Consulting your pediatrician is important in any questionable dietary decisions. Generally, women do not need to avoid many foods while breastfeeding. They do need to eat a healthy and diverse diet for themselves and their babies.

Taking in enough fluids is important to the breastfeeding mother. She should "drink to thirst" and try to have a glass of water or beverage when or after she feeds her baby. Everyone's fluid needs will be different. Approximately 8-12 cups of water a day is sometimes suggested for pregnancy intake, and even more is needed when breastfeeding. If any signs of dehydration occur, dry skin, muscle cramps, headaches, dizziness, or dark urine she needs to increase her fluid intake.

As a new dad, you can play a crucial role in supporting the breastfeeding mother by assisting with meal planning and preparation for your family. This involves helping to grocery shop, cook meals, or even prepping snacks for her to grab on the go. By sharing the responsibility for meal planning, you can alleviate some stress the new mother may feel.

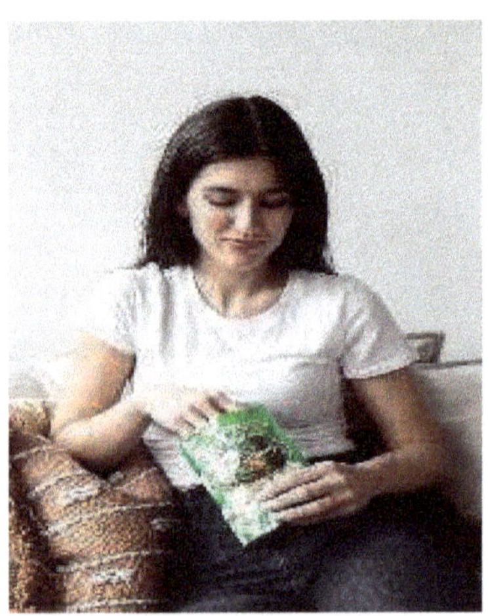

"The whole human world is born from the womb of mothers, and if we can't make the motherly act of breastfeeding free from stigma in such a world, then it's an insult to our very existence as a species."

-Abhijit Naskar

Chapter 3
Advocating for the Breastfeeding Mother in Social and Professional Settings & Laws on Breastfeeding

Advocating for breastfeeding mothers in social and professional settings is crucial. It is important to understand that breastfeeding mothers may face challenges when trying to breastfeed in public or while at work, and it is the responsibility of both partners to help advocate for their rights and create a supportive environment.

In social settings, new dads can educate friends and family about the benefits of breastfeeding for both mother and baby. By sharing this knowledge, new dads can help create a supportive and understanding environment for the breastfeeding mother, making it easier for her to breastfeed anywhere without feeling judged or uncomfortable.

In professional settings, new dads can support breastfeeding mothers by standing up for their right to pump at work. It is important to familiarize oneself with current laws and regulations that protect the rights of breastfeeding mothers in the workplace. Work with your partner and the employer to create a safe and private space for pumping her milk to maintain her supply and collect milk for later. By advocating along with the breastfeeding mother in the workplace, new dads help ensure that she is able to continue breastfeeding while maintaining her career.

Laws of Breastfeeding

It is legal to Breastfeed in the United States. "All fifty states, the District of Columbia, Puerto Rico and the Virgin Islands have laws that specifically allow women to breastfeed in any public or private location." Aug 26, 2021, www.ncsl.org>ueaptu>breastfeeding

In most states, "these laws also prohibit anyone from interfering with a woman who is breastfeeding, including asking her to move to a different location or cover-up." "The Patient Protection and Affordable Care Act (ACA), which was signed into law in 2010, includes a provision that requires employers to provide reasonable break time for an employee to express breastmilk for her nursing child for one year after the child's birth. Employers must also provide a private place, other than a bathroom, for the employee to express breast milk." www.usbreastfeeding.org/,
www.ncs.org/reseach/health/breastfeeding-state-laws.aspx,
www.womenshealth.gov/breastfeeding/learningbreastfeed/breastfeeding-and-law

<u>If you travel outside of the U.S., please check, the current laws where you plan to travel.</u>

Overall, advocating for the breastfeeding mother in social and professional settings is an essential part of supporting her breastfeeding journey. It is important to be a strong advocate for the breastfeeding mother, both in public and at work, to ensure that she is able to breastfeed successfully and comfortably.

"Children are not a distraction from more important work. They are the most important work."

-C.S. Lewis

Chapter 4
Mechanics of Breastfeeding, How and When to Feed Your Baby

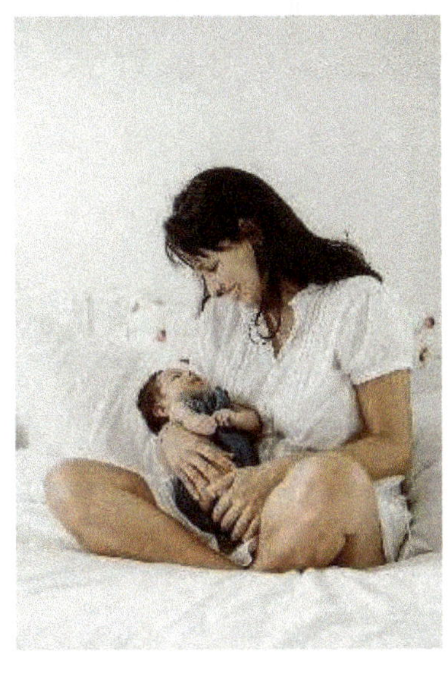

Learning about the mechanics of breastfeeding is an essential aspect for new parents. Understanding how breastfeeding works, including proper positioning and latch and when to feed your baby, can make a significant difference in the success of breastfeeding.

Proper positioning is key to ensuring that both mother and baby are comfortable and able to nurse effectively. New dads can help their partner find a comfortable position for breastfeeding. Bringing her pillows for support, assisting in adjusting the baby's position to achieve a proper latch, and helping keep the baby awake can be very helpful.

The photo on this page shows a baby with a wide latch.

Baby has a lot of breast tissue in its mouth. This will be more comfortable for the mother and release more milk for the baby.

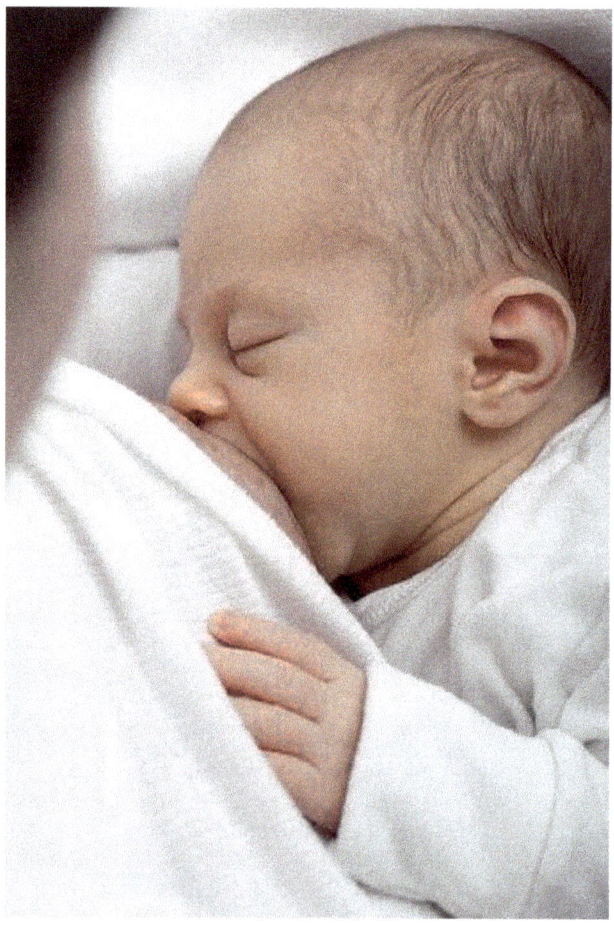

Assisting with Proper Positioning and Latch

To assist with proper positioning, it's important to help the mother find a comfortable and relaxed position for feeding. This may involve using pillows or a nursing pillow to support the baby at the breast level. Make sure to have rolled receiving blankets or pillows for Mom to rest her arms on and one for behind her back if needed. Encourage the mother to bring the baby to the breast, rather than leaning over to the baby, to prevent strain on her back and shoulders. Look to see if she is tensing her shoulders up, and if so, mention that she can take a deep breath and relax her shoulders. The baby's stomach should face the mother's body, "tummy to tummy," so the baby's face faces the breast. Again, the baby should also be level with the mother's breast, use a pillow or nursing pillow to raise the baby to this level. At first, when the baby's neck isn't strong enough, support around their head ear to ear without pushing on the back of their head. This can be achieved by mom putting her thumb near one ear and other fingers near the other ear. The cross-cradle hold and football holds are a few of the positions that are good for new mothers to try. On the next page is a graphic of some breastfeeding holds. Any position will work as long as the mother is comfortable, has control of the baby, and the baby has a deep latch and is comfortable.

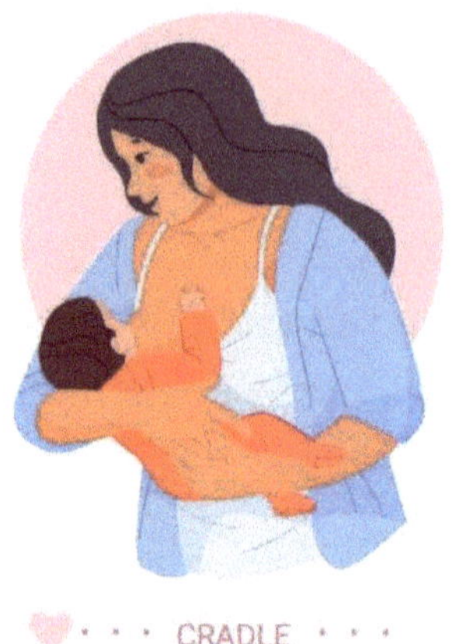

♥ · · · CRADLE · · ·

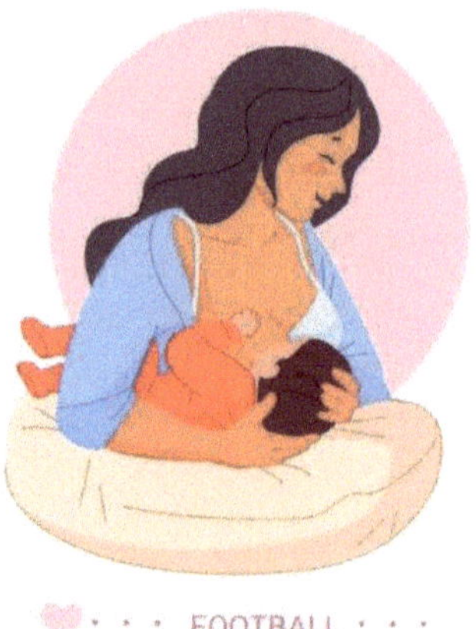

♥ · · · FOOTBALL · · ·

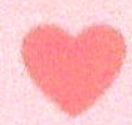 ♥ **BREASTFEEDING** ♥ 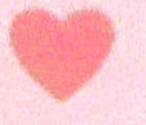

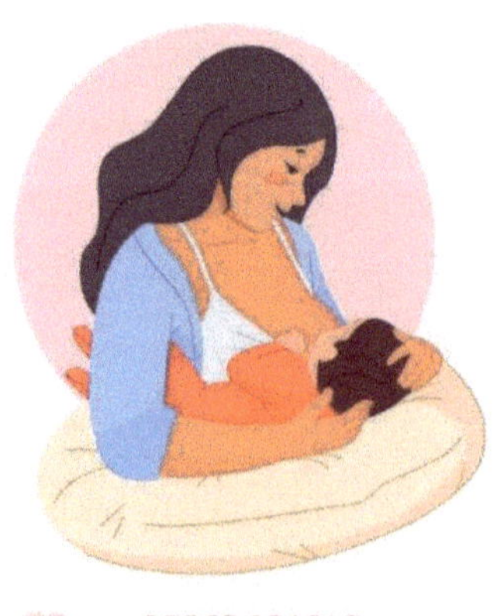

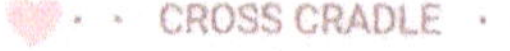

♥ · · CROSS CRADLE · ·

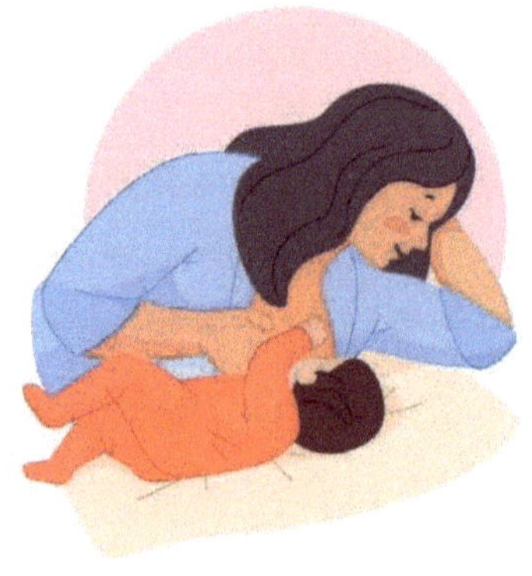

♥ · · · SIDE-LYING · · ·

If the baby falls asleep before the feeding is finished you can help by rubbing their feet or body to help wake them to eat. The baby may need to be taken out of their blanket to wake them up for a feeding. Mom can also massage or gently squeeze her breast to help the milk come out quicker.

It's very important for the baby to have what is referred to as a "wide or deep latch." Wait for the baby to open wide, like a yawn, and quickly pull them towards the mother's breast so that they get a large mouthful of breast tissue. They need to latch on around the nipple, on the areola, not on the nipple! This will take patience and practice. All involved are learning how to do this. It can take multiple tries, but it is worth mom's comfort to do this properly. If the baby has a "shallow latch," not a deep latch, put a clean finger in between the baby's mouth and the mother's breast to break the suction first to remove the baby and try again.

If the mother's breasts are engorged or have enlarged during milk production, it can be difficult for the baby to latch. Mothers can try to either hand express or pump some milk first to soften the area around the nipple/areola. She can also try to press the fluid inside the breast, around the nipple/areola area, back and away right before the baby tries to latch.

Remember, breastfeeding is a learned skill for both mother and baby. Multiple attempts are normal, and it's okay to seek help from a lactation consultant if needed.

Nursing Station

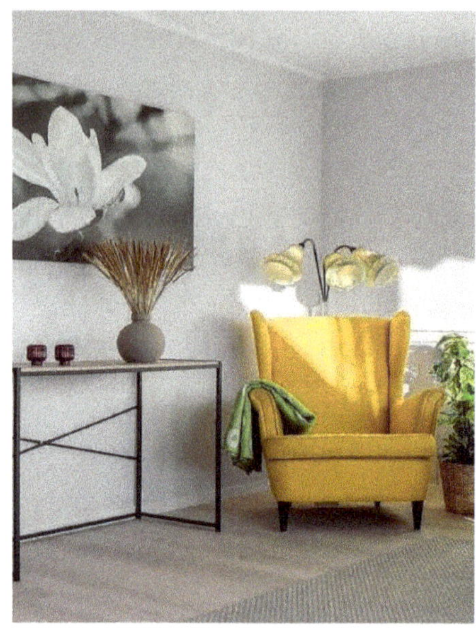

It is a good idea to create at least one area in the house for breastfeeding or a "Nursing Station". A comfortable chair, a table for a glass of water, pillows and blankets, nipple balm, burping cloths, and hair ties are some things that should be conveniently available. Whatever makes the mom comfortable to feed the baby, have nearby. It is also good to have a footrest to elevate her feet.

By assisting with making the mother comfortable and ensuring she has everything she needs when feeding the baby, you are promoting a caring and loving relationship between you, the mother and your baby. Your support and encouragement can make a significant difference in the breastfeeding journey, so don't underestimate the impact you can have as a new dad.

Managing Common Challenges and Troubleshooting Issues

Breastfeeding can be a rewarding experience for both mother and baby, but it can also come with its fair share of challenges. As a new dad, it's important to be prepared for any hurdles that may arise and know how to troubleshoot them effectively.

One of the most common challenges that new mothers face when breastfeeding is nipple pain or discomfort. This can be caused by improper latch, engorgement, or other issues. New dads can support their partners by helping them troubleshoot these challenges, whether it's seeking help from a lactation consultant or trying different nursing positions. Your lactation consultant or health care provider may suggest using mom's own breast milk or ultra-pure lanolin to apply to her nipples. These can help relieve some discomfort and are both fine for the baby to ingest. Gel pads are also available to cool and relieve discomfort. Another possibility is that the baby has "tongue-tie" or ankyloglossia. This needs to be confirmed by your pediatrician. Lastly, check for a skin yeast infection around the nipple area. This could also be a cause of discomfort and needs to be addressed. By understanding common breastfeeding challenges and how to address them, new dads can provide valuable support to their breastfeeding partner and help them navigate any issues that may arise. If you aren't sure and need extra assistance, call your lactation consultant or doctor for guidance.

Another common issue that was mentioned above is engorgement. This occurs when the breasts become overly full of milk, leading to discomfort and potential difficulty for the baby to latch on. To help alleviate engorgement, encourage the breastfeeding mother to nurse frequently and ensure that she is wearing a comfortable and supportive bra. You can also assist by mentioning to the mom to gently massage the breasts or apply warm compresses to help relieve the pressure.

Blocked ducts are another common issue that can occur during breastfeeding. If you notice that the breastfeeding mother is experiencing pain, redness, or a hard lump in her breast, it may be a sign of a blocked duct. To help resolve this issue, encourage her to nurse frequently on the affected side, apply warm compresses, and she can gently massage the area to help release the blockage. It's also important to ensure that she is getting enough rest and staying hydrated to help prevent further blockages from occurring.

Mastitis is a more serious issue that can occur if a blocked duct is not resolved promptly. This condition is characterized by inflammation and infection of the breast tissue, leading to symptoms such as fever, chills, and flu-like symptoms. If you suspect that the breastfeeding mother may have mastitis, it's important to seek medical attention immediately. Encourage her to continue nursing on the affected side, as this can help to clear the infection and prevent further complications.

Remember to call your doctor or lactation consultant if you have questions. By being proactive and informed, you can help to ensure that breastfeeding is a positive and successful experience.

The World Health Organization recommends "Early initiation of breastfeeding within 1 hour of birth."

****

The American Academy of Pediatrics recommends "Exclusive breastfeeding for about the first six months, with continued breastfeeding along with introducing appropriate complementary foods for up to 2 years of age or longer."

Chapter 5
Feeding Your Baby & Hunger Cues
Feeding your Baby

Your infant needs to be fed whenever they are hungry or at least 8-12 times every 24 hours for about the first month of life. That can be every two hours if they need it. This is around the clock at first, they have been fed 24/7 in the womb and have never felt hunger before. They need this nutrition for their rapid growth. Their stomachs are very small at first, around the size of a small marble or cherry. Mom's body will be able to produce the amount of milk colostrum at first that the baby needs. As long as she is consistent with nursing her baby when they are hungry or 8-12 times every 24 hours, her body will know to start producing the milk that the baby needs. The suckling of the baby and the removal of milk tells her body how much milk to make. If she skips a feeding, her body will make less. Breastfeeding is a "supply/demand" system. The mother's milk supply depends on how often she feeds or pumps. The more milk that is removed, the more milk her body will make.

The time immediately after your baby is born is referred to as the "Golden Hour," which actually can be up to three hours. This is a wonderful time for special mother-baby bonding. The baby will most likely be awake, not fussy and want to nurse. This is the transitional period of time from being in utero to acclimating to the outside world with their mother and father. If possible, uninterrupted skin-to-skin with the mother, until the baby shows signs of hunger and begins their first feeding is ideally what you would like to happen.

Skin to Skin or Kangaroo care is important for your baby. This is when you place your infant, diaper only, on your bare chest, their ear to your chest, and cover their back with a blanket. There are many benefits to making this a part of your early parenting, and both moms and dads can do this. When mom does skin to skin with the baby, her body will warm up to what the baby needs. The baby will also be in a perfect position to move right into a feeding when you notice their hunger cues. Some of the benefits of kangaroo care are improved breastfeeding, warming of the baby, stabilizing their heartbeat and breathing, less crying, and increased weight gain. They may even be able to hear your heartbeat, breathing sounds, and can feel the motion of your chest moving up and down. It's a beneficial and beautiful way to spend quality time with your new baby.

The first milk is called "colostrum" or sometimes called "liquid gold." This very concentrated milk has everything the baby needs and in small amounts for their small stomach. By days 3-5, colostrum will start transitioning, and more milk will be produced, causing mom's breasts to become very full. This stage may be uncomfortable for the mom at first. She may need to express some milk first to make it easier for the baby to latch on. If you need extra help at this point, ask your lactation consultant for assistance. As the baby grows, the milk will transition to "Mature Milk" around 10-15 days after birth. Your baby will transition to about 7-9 feedings a day at around 1 to 2 months old. Around 6 months old, they will nurse about 6 times a day and around a year old, nursing can drop to 4 times a day. There will be times when they seem hungry constantly and need to be fed more. The baby's growth phases will contribute to the amount of food they need.

Because of this extremely active schedule, the baby's mom should try to sleep when the baby sleeps!

Hunger Cues

Your baby will give you signs when they are hungry. The signs could be tongue movements, head moving from side to side, hands to their mouth, lip smacking, opening their mouth and more. Every baby will have their own signs. As soon as you notice these, get the baby to latch deeply as soon as possible. At first, remember, it can take a few tries to get a deep latch. It is very normal to try multiple times at first to get a deep, comfortable latch. You don't want to wait until the baby cries to feed them because it will be frustrating to get your baby latched on at this point.

The baby below is showing the hunger cue of hands in the mouth.

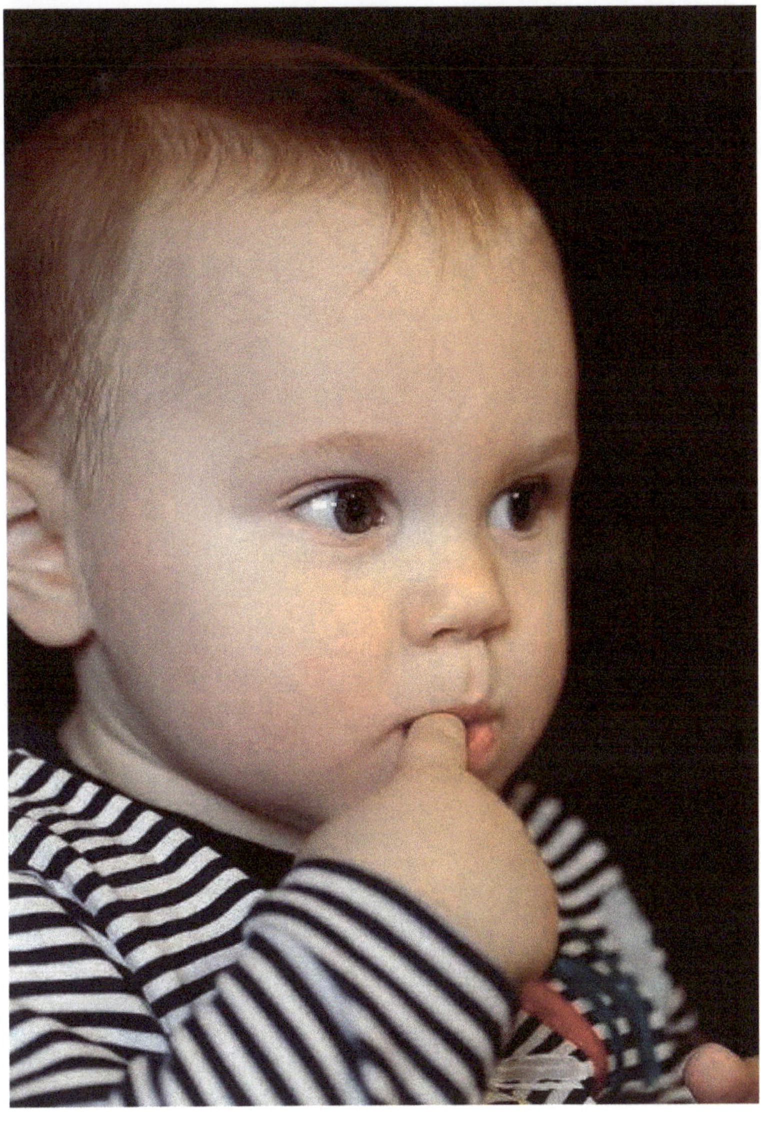

This baby is showing a hunger cue. Open mouth, turning head towards the breast.

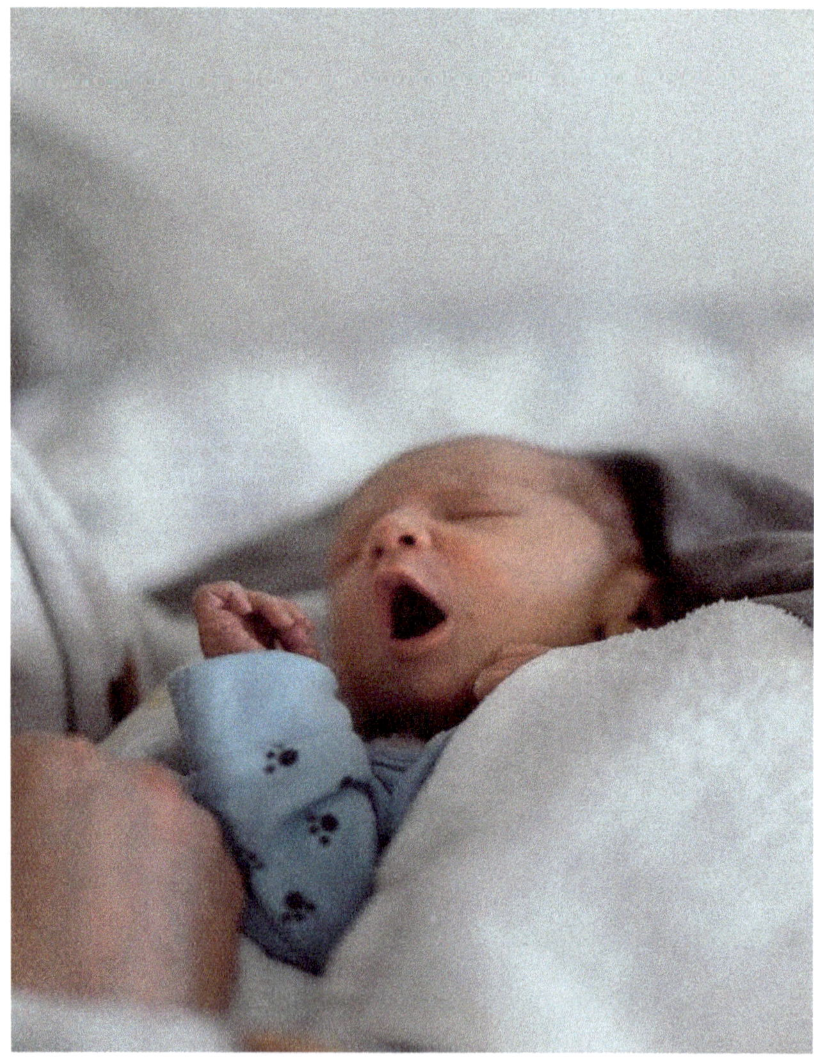

A few things to advocate for right after the birth

-Place the baby skin-to-skin or Kangaroo Care on the mom's chest.

-Ideally, have a first feeding within 1.5 hours after the birth.

- The new mother may be exhausted or groggy and might need either your help, a nurse or a lactation consultant to help the baby get a nice wide latch for their feeding. The baby should latch around the nipple, not on the nipple. A shallow latch will contribute to soreness for the mom and less milk for the baby.

"Love is not just about finding the right partner; it is also about being the right partner."

-Unknown

Chapter 6
Creating a Supportive Environment, Baby Blues, Postpartum Depression, & Reframing Your Lives

Creating a Supportive Environment

Providing emotional, physical and household support for the breastfeeding mother is a crucial aspect of being a new dad. Breastfeeding can be a challenging and emotionally taxing experience for many mothers, so it's important for new dads to be understanding, patient, and encouraging throughout the process. One of the best ways to provide emotional support is to listen to the mother's feelings and concerns without judgment. Encourage her to express her emotions and be there to offer comfort and reassurance.

New mothers will fall on a scale between being very comfortable breastfeeding to being very shy and reserved about this new experience. There may be physical and emotional obstacles for the two of you to work on together. How women feel about breastfeeding is very personal.

The United States and some other cultures sexualize breasts, and seeing women breastfeed at home, in the media or in public may not happen often. This can contribute to the mother and you feeling awkward and uncomfortable at first. In the 1950's when formula became readily available it was thought to be just like breastmilk. Breastfeeding was seen as only for those who couldn't afford formula and was discouraged by medical practitioners and the media at that time. With current knowledge about the benefits of breastfeeding, parents and healthcare providers now see this as the optimal choice for those who are able. As more women get back to breastfeeding in the States, this will become more common for everyone.

It's very important for new dads to help moms with emotional and physical needs and also with household responsibilities. This includes helping with chores, taking care of other children, and offering to cook meals or run errands. By lightening the mother's load, new dads can help alleviate stress and allow her to focus on breastfeeding and bonding with the baby.

By working together as a team, new parents can navigate the challenges of breastfeeding and create a positive and nurturing environment for the entire family.

Baby Blues & Postpartum Depression

Many new moms can experience postpartum 'baby blues' after childbirth." A few days after childbirth, a new mother may experience mood swings, crying spells, sleep problems and or anxiety. This can last up to a few weeks.

Some new mothers experience a more severe and longer-lasting type of depression called "Postpartum Depression." Some symptoms of this are longer-lasting and more severe depressed mood or mood swings, crying, withdrawal, inability to bond with the baby, and more. If you see signs of this, call the mother's physician immediately. This is a treatable condition.

Very <u>rarely,</u> a condition called Postpartum Psychosis can occur. These symptoms can include confusion, hallucinations, delusions, foreseeing an ominous future, and even attempts to harm herself or the child. This condition can be life-threatening and requires immediate treatment.

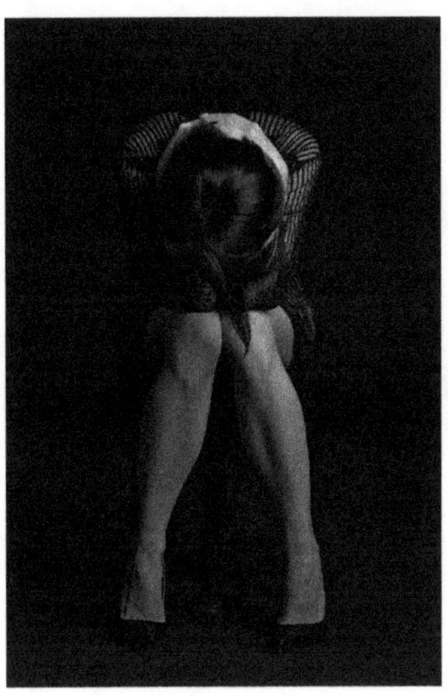

Re-framing Your Lives

Navigating potential challenges or conflicts in the family can be an unsettling task, especially for new parents who are still adjusting to their new roles and responsibilities. When it comes to supporting a breastfeeding mother, it is important for new dads to understand that breastfeeding is a team effort and that their encouragement is crucial in ensuring success.

Once you are home with your new child, life will be very different from what it was before. It can be the best and possibly the most challenging time of your life. Re-framing, modifying or seeing things from a different perspective can help soften the stress of these changes. If you find yourself challenged and upset about the changes happening, try to notice these upsetting thoughts and do your best to find the positive things going on and focus on those. Work on managing your expectations of each other. Instead of seeing some of the new changes as problems, try to see them as challenges. An example of re-framing something would be, "I need 8 straight hours of sleep" re-frame to "I will try to get 8 hours of sleep by sleeping whenever it's possible." Rising to the occasion is going to be necessary, along with patience and understanding.

Communication will be key. It is important for new parents to openly discuss their feelings, concerns, and needs with each other. You will have to find common ground and work together as a team. By maintaining open and honest communication, new parents can address any issues that may arise and find solutions that work for both. Having Empathy, or trying your best to understand what your partner is going through, is very important, especially at this changing time in your life.

If you start to feel overwhelmed, take a breath, try to reframe the situation or ask for more help. Remember, your lack of sleep will contribute to your overall demeanor. Nap, if possible, when the baby naps!

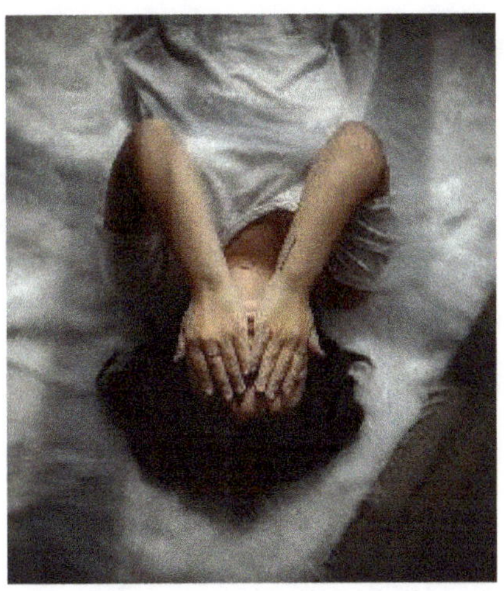

Overall, navigating potential challenges or conflicts in the family requires patience, understanding, and a willingness to work together as a team. By supporting each other, communicating effectively, and managing expectations, new parents can overcome any obstacles that may arise and create a supportive environment for the breastfeeding mother and the baby.

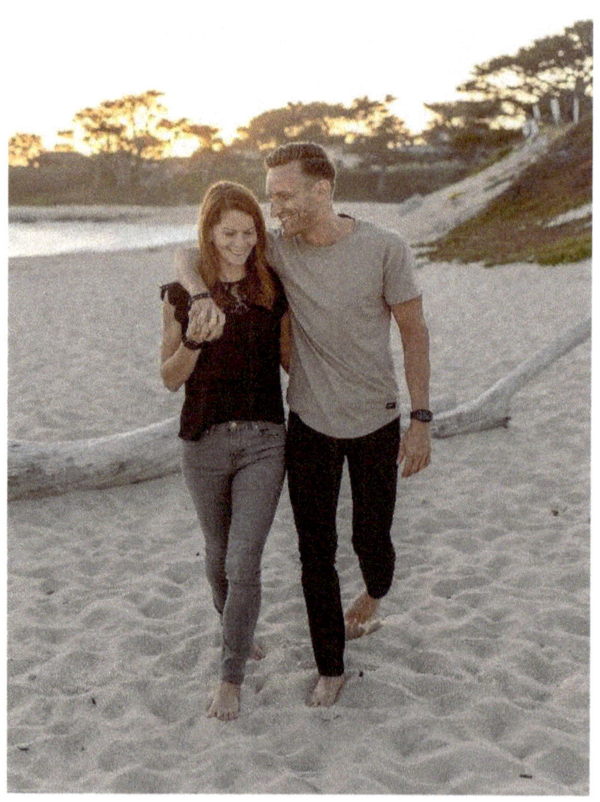

"To be a good parent, you need to take care of
yourself so that you can have the physical and
emotional energy to take care of your family."

- Parentselfcare.com

Chapter 7
Self-Care for the Breastfeeding Mother
Understanding the Importance of Self-Care

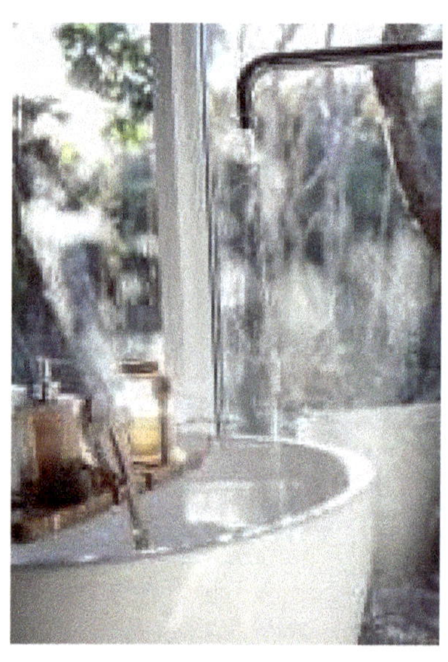

Self-care is a crucial aspect of supporting a breastfeeding mother, as it allows her to prioritize her own well-being in order to better care for her baby. As a new dad, it is important to recognize that taking care of oneself is not selfish but rather essential for maintaining physical and mental health. By understanding the importance of self-care, you can better support the breastfeeding mother in your life and create a nurturing environment for both her and your baby.

One of the key benefits of self-care for a breastfeeding mother is the ability to recharge and replenish her energy levels. Breastfeeding can be physically demanding, and it is important for the mother to take time to rest and recuperate in order to maintain her milk supply and overall health. By encouraging her to prioritize self-care, you are helping to ensure that she has the energy and stamina to continue breastfeeding for as long as she desires.

In addition to physical benefits, self-care also plays a crucial role in supporting the mental and emotional well-being of a breastfeeding mother. The demands of caring for a newborn can be overwhelming, and it is common for mothers to experience feelings of stress, anxiety, and exhaustion. By encouraging self-care practices such as meditation, exercise, or taking breaks when needed, you can help the mother to reduce feelings of overwhelm and maintain a positive mindset.

Ultimately, self-care is important not only for the well-being of the breastfeeding mother but also for the entire family dynamic. By understanding the importance of self-care for your partner and yourself you are contributing to a positive and nurturing environment for your baby to thrive. Remember, self-care is not a luxury but a necessity for maintaining health and happiness during parenting and breastfeeding.

"Pumping breastmilk provides expressed breastmilk for the times a mother will be away from her baby. For when she goes back to work, to school, is running errands or taking time for self-care. This not only gives you flexibility to feed the baby at a later time, but increases milk production."

-H. M. Scott

Chapter 8
Pumping and Storing Breastmilk
Understanding the Role of Pumping

Pumping breastmilk is an important aspect of breastfeeding that allows milk to be stored. The milk can then be used by the dad or others to feed the baby. Pumping also allows the breastfeeding mother to have flexibility in her feeding routine and enables her to continue breastfeeding even when she is away from her baby. Pumping is not necessary if a mother produces enough milk and doesn't want to store extra milk for others to take over some breast milk feedings.

One of the key benefits of pumping is that it helps to maintain the mother's milk supply. By regularly pumping breastmilk, the breastfeeding mother can ensure that she has a steady supply of milk for her baby, even when she is unable to breastfeed directly.

Discuss which pump to purchase and the best ways to safely store the milk with your doctor or lactation Consultant. Check with your insurance company to see if they cover breast pumps. New dads can support the pumping process by helping to set up and clean the pump, as well as by assisting with storing the breastmilk.

Managing common challenges together that may arise during pumping, such as low milk supply or discomfort, is another way you can support the mother. By troubleshooting these issues together and finding solutions, you can help make the pumping experience more successful and less stressful for her. Read through the instructions that came with the pump and make sure the flange size is correct. Additionally, you can assist with storing the pumped breastmilk in clean, labeled containers and ensuring that it is stored properly in the refrigerator or freezer. Understanding the role of pumping and storing breastmilk is another way to be a supportive partner.

A benefit of pumping is that dads/fathers/partners can participate in feeding the baby.

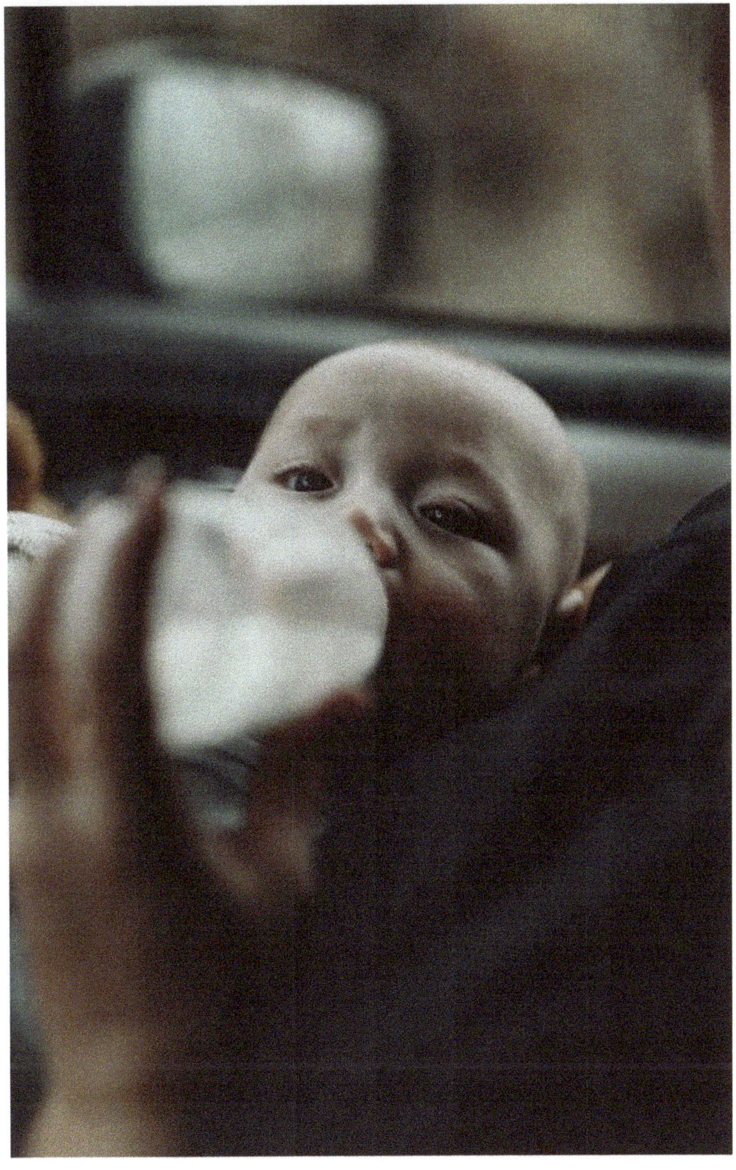

"We made a wish, and two came true." - anonymous

"If you think my hands are full, you should see my heart." -Unknown

Chapter 9
Twins and Multiples

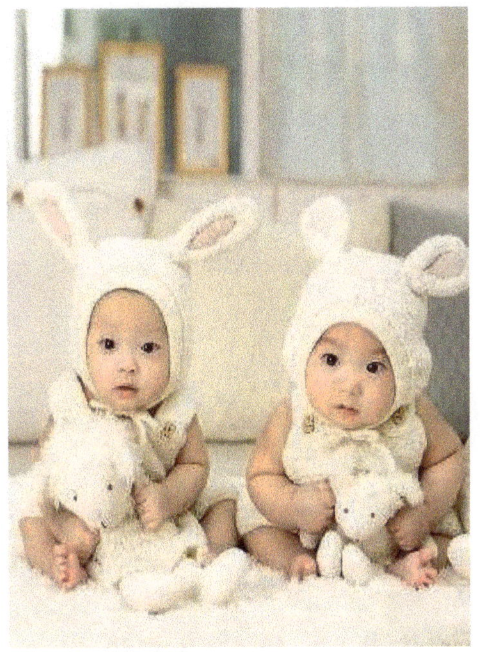

Extra Support is needed for a mother of twins or multiples. If the new mother chooses to breastfeed, in most cases, her body will produce enough milk for all of her babies if they are removing enough milk from her." Mothers of twins consistently released twice the volume of milk as mothers of singletons. Mothers of triplets were capable of producing up to a remarkable volume of more than 3 liters/day when the infants were aged 2.5 months." https://www.ncbi.nlm.nih.gov>pmc

Lack of sleep and new parenthood can be twice as challenging for parents of twins. Freedom of choice on how to feed multiples is very important. Getting the babies fed is the priority. Any amount of breastmilk is beneficial for babies. If Breastfeeding is your choice, make sure you have all of the support you need. Try to find a group, club or other parents with multiples for support and information. Contact a lactation consultant and your pediatrician with any questions or concerns.

It is important for parents to feel confident in any way they choose to feed their children, and primarily important for the children to be fed. The following graphic has a picture of some of the positions a mother of twins can try.

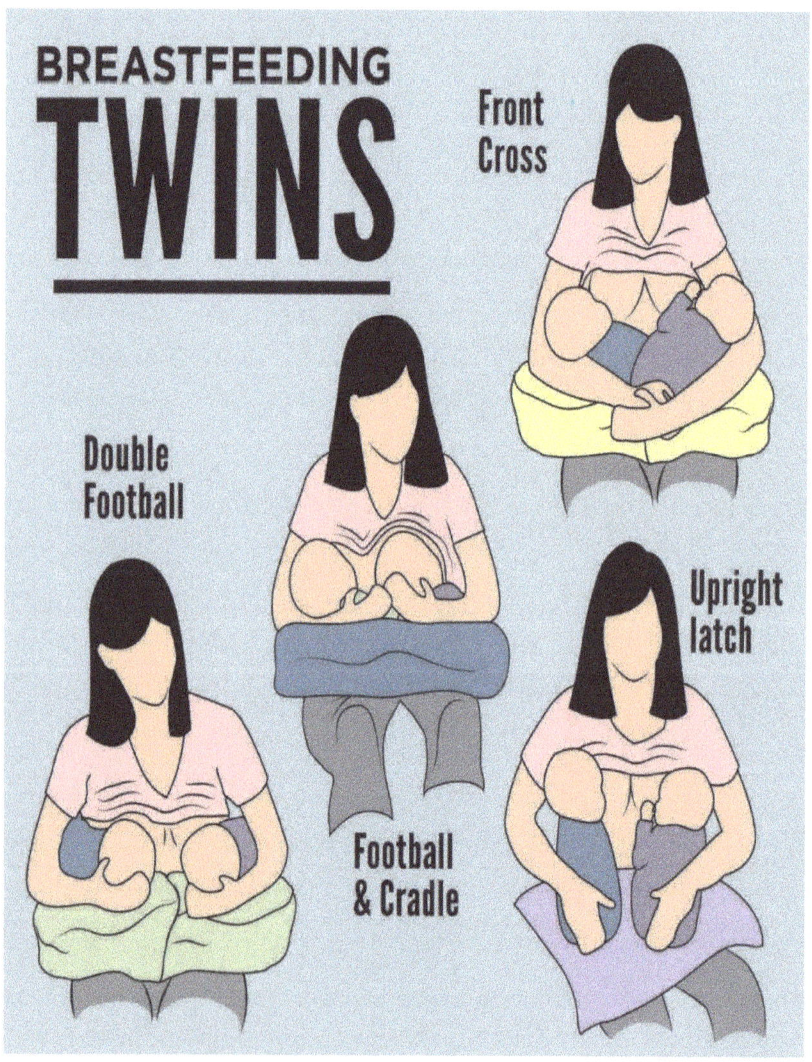

"The most important thing a father can do for his children is to love their mother."

-Theodore Hesburgh

***

"To the new parents, don't forget to be kind to yourselves and to each other. You are both new to this. You will both have moments of insecurity and overwhelm. So, talk to each other, be supportive, be proud of your partner and encourage them. There is no one way to parent, so learn and guide each other so you can both be the very best parents you can be."

-Proudhappymama.com

Chapter 10
Conclusion & Resources

Studies do show that men and partners are instrumental in working with moms to ensure the best possible outcome with breastfeeding. "A father's knowledge and attitude are fundamental in beginning and maintaining breastfeeding. He has the most critical role in helping women with parenting and feeding their babies." Cureus, 2022 Oct; 14. Educating fathers/dads/partners can be a tremendous help to mothers and infants learning how to breastfeed and to help promote and destigmatize breastfeeding for all.

As a new dad, understanding the resources and support networks available for breastfeeding mothers is essential in providing the best support for your partner. Breastfeeding can be a challenging journey, but with the right tools and information, you can help make the experience more enjoyable for both mother and baby. By exploring the various resources and support networks that exist, you can ensure that your partner has access to the help she needs to succeed in her breastfeeding journey.

Creating a supportive environment for the breastfeeding mother is crucial in ensuring her success. This includes providing emotional support, helping with household tasks, and making sure she has access to nutritious meals and snacks. By being there for your partner and offering your support in any way you can, you help make her breastfeeding experience more enjoyable and successful.

Resources

<u>La Leche League International,</u>

Dedicated to supporting and educating mothers about breastfeeding, including local La Leche League groups. https://llli.org>breastfeeding-info

<u>Breastfeeding Helpline</u>

800-944-9662

The National Women's Health and Breastfeeding Helpline offers breastfeeding information anytime between 9 am and 6 pm Eastern, Monday through Friday, in English or Spanish.

<u>Kellymom.com</u>

A website to provide evidence-based information on breastfeeding and parenting

<u>Lactation Consultants</u>

Ask your hospital, Obstetrician, Pediatrician or midwife for the name of a lactation Consultant. Or go to the IBCLC Certification Registry.

<u>There are many resources online. Please make sure you use reputable sites that are also up to date.</u>

Helpful Tips

Signs, Charts and Lists you may need

1. Dads or partners need to play "bouncer" in the hospital when moms and babies are learning to breastfeed. This is a critical time for new mothers to have privacy while learning to feed their babies. You may want to find a lactation consultant or nurse who can offer guidance and reassurance. The idea is to post a sign outside the door for visitors stating,

"Baby is learning to eat; please wait for a little while to visit. You can text me to let me know you are here, and I will let you know when we are ready for visitors."

2. When you arrive home, you can make a "To-Do" list to post on your refrigerator or somewhere where all can see it. List household chores such as starting the laundry, folding the laundry, cleaning the dishes, walking the dog, picking up groceries, etc. If family or friends come to visit when you are resting for feeding the baby, and they ask how they can help, you can suggest that it would be helpful to do anything on your list.

3. Search online for an easy-to-use breastfeeding log to keep track of when the baby eats, which side they start on, and how long they ate. You will also need a chart to track their poops and pees. This will help ensure that your baby is eating enough. Your pediatrician will probably also want to see these charts when you come in for appointments. There are some charts that have places to track all of these things, or you can create your own.

Important Contacts

Pediatrician

Lactation Consultant

OBGYN

Primary Doctors

Other medical professionals and important contacts

Questions to ask Medical Professionals

Test Your Knowledge

1. **Which of the following are in breast milk but not in infant formula?**
   A. Antibodies
   B. Growth Factors
   C. Anti-Allergies
      A. & C.
      B. All of the above
      C. None of the above

2. **Which of the following are the benefits of Breastfeeding for the mother?**
      A. Reduces some cancer risks
      B. Helps uterus contract back to pre-pregnancy size
      C. Stress relief hormone
   A & B
   A & C
   All of the above

3. **If a breastfeeding mother gets a cold, the baby will receive antibodies from the breast milk to help fight this cold.**
   True or False

4. **Breastfeeding can lower the risk of SIDS (Sudden Infant Death Syndrome)**
   True or False

5. **How often does a newborn infant have to eat every 24 hours?**

Answers to Test Your Knowledge

1. All of the above

2. All of the above

3. True

4. True

5. 8-12 feedings every 24 hours

Notes:

Notes:

Notes:

Notes:

Notes:

Notes:

References

AAP (American Academy of Pediatrics) Breastfeeding and the Use of Human Milk. Pediatrics 115:496-506

Academy of Breastfeeding Medicine. Breastfeeding Medicine 3:38-43

Ata Paediatr, 2019 Jul: 108(7) : 1192-1204

Bergman, N. Kangaroo Mother Care; Presentation at La Leche League Internationals 29th Seminar for Physicians on Breastfeeding, Chicago, IL.
https;//Internationalbreastfeedingjournal.November 29, 2009
https://www.pregnancybirthbaby.org.au
cdc.gov,johnshopkinsmedicine.org, https://hipkinsmedicine.org, Breast Milk is Best Cureus, 2022 Oct:14(10):e30363. online Oct 16

Le Leche League International site, LLLI.org

National Conference of State Legislatures-
https://www.ncsl.org/research/health/breastfeeding-state-laws.aspx National Institutes of Health
www.ncbi.nlm.nih.gov>pmc
www.ncsl.org>ueaptu>breastfeeding www.nichd.nih.gov>bene ts of breastfeeding

Once on Women's Health-U.S. Department of Health & Human

Services
https://www.womenshealth.gov/breastfeeding/learning-breastfeed/breastfeeding-and-lae
https://www.who.int/new(Jun 9,2021)

Unicef https://www.who.int/new

United States Breastfeeding Committee-
https://www.usbreastfeeding.org/

Photos and graphics licensed from Adobe and Designer

About the Author

Mae Scott lives in Charlotte, North Carolina with her family. Her interests related to this book topic are teaching, reading, continual education, family dynamics, and child development.

Mae earned a BA from University of Delaware in Psychology with concentrations in Child Development, Communications, and Design. She completed her Lactation Consultant Education and Internship at Novant's Presbyterian Hospital in Charlotte, North Carolina. She has been a member of the International Board of Lactation Consultants for 10 years, and is a certified IBCLC. She was an educator for Novant's Presbyterian Hospitals, Women's Health Education Department in Charlotte, North Carolina. There she taught Lactation and both premature and full-term Infant Massage. She also worked for Inova Hospital System near Washington, D.C. teaching Lactation and Infant Massage. Her previous career as a Dental Hygienist, R.D.H. gave her knowledge and insight into how oral anatomy and function influences breastfeeding.

Combining her education and experiences, she hopes her writing will make a positive impact in many lives.

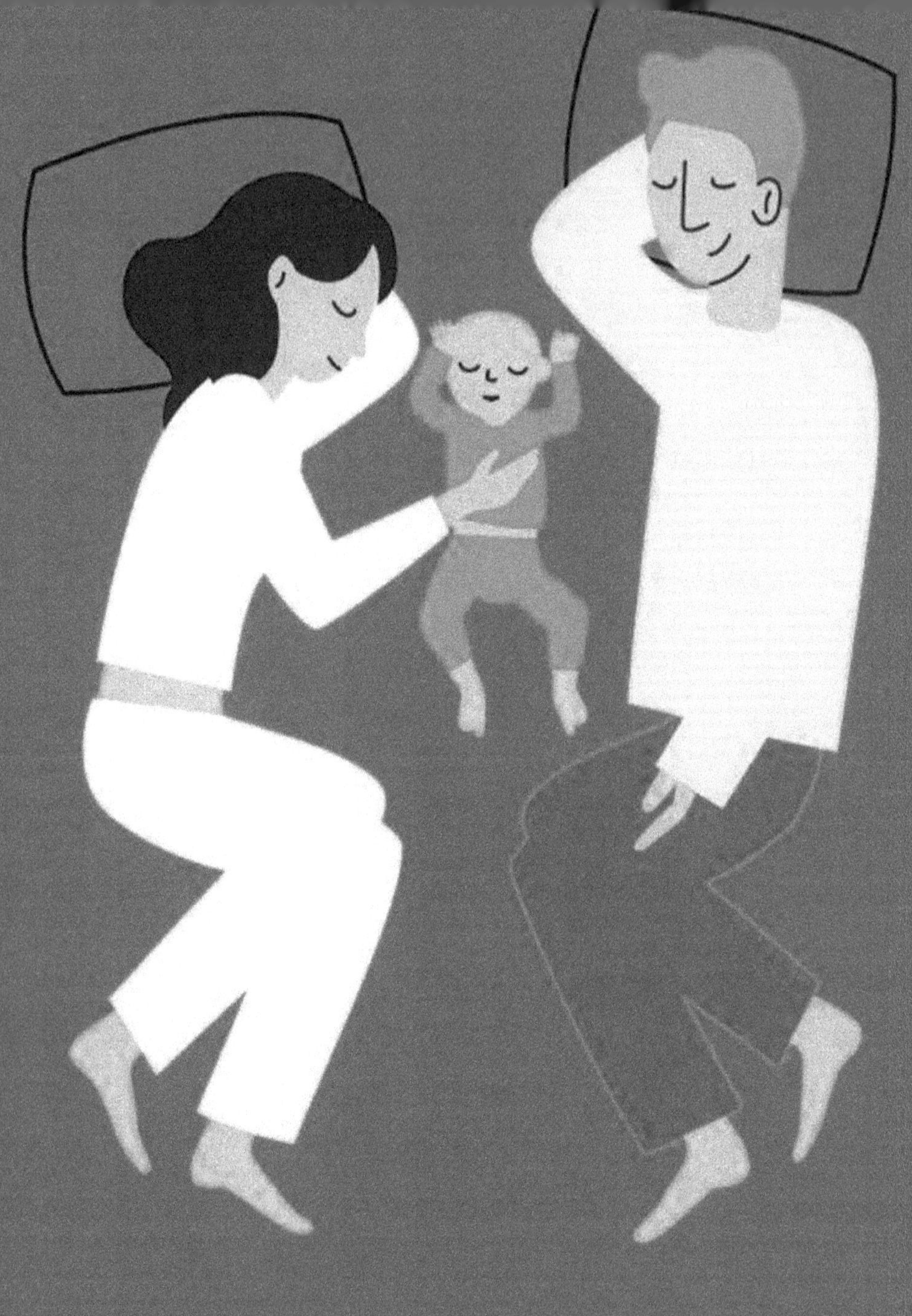

Bed-sharing is a controversial topic. You must check with your pediatrician. La Leche league International has released, "Safe Sleep 7." This is a guide to safer bed-sharing.